SHINGLES

THINGS YOU SHOULD KNOW

(QUESTIONS AND ANSWERS)

By Rumi Michael Leigh

Introduction

I would like to thank and congratulate you for purchasing this book, " *Shingles, things you should know (questions and answers)*" series.

This book will help you understand, revise and have a good general knowledge and keywords of shingles and its effect on the body.

Thanks again for purchasing this book, I hope you enjoy it!

Table of Contents

Section 1

1) What is shingles?

- Shingles is a viral disease that causes painful rash.

2) Can shingles cause pain without the presence of rash?

- Yes, shingles can cause pain without the presence of rash.

3) What virus causes shingles?

- The virus that causes shingles is the varicella zoster virus.

4) Shingles is also called?

- Shingles is also called herpes zoster or zoster.

5) Can shingles occur anywhere in the body?

- Yes, shingles can occur anywhere in the body.

6) Does shingles usually appear on both sides of the body?

- No, shingles does not usually appear on both sides of the body. It usually appears on one side of the body.

7) Can a person have shingles more than one time?

- Yes, a person can have shingles more than one time.

8) Is there a cure for shingles?

- No, there is no cure for shingles.

9) Can the shingles virus remain dormant for life in a person?

- Yes, the shingles virus can remain dormant for life in a person.

10) What is dormant?

- Dormant means inactive.

Section 2

1) How can shingles be prevented?

- Shingles can be prevented using a shingles vaccine.

2) How can a person prevent the spreading of shingles virus?

- A person can prevent the spreading of shingles virus by covering and avoid touching the rash, having a good hygiene by washing the hands several times daily and avoiding contact with people until the rash dries out.

3) Can shingles be treated?

- Yes, shingles can be treated.

4) When should the treatment of shingles begin?

- The treatment of shingles should begin as soon as possible.

5) What are the treatments for shingles?

- The treatments for shingles include antiviral drugs, painkillers, local anesthetic, anti-inflammation drugs, numbing creams, antihistamines, and antidepressants.

6) How long does it take for shingles to clear up?

- It takes about 2 to 4 weeks for shingles to clear up.

7) Is shingles a common condition?

- Yes, shingles is a common condition.

8) Is shingles life-threatening?

- No, shingles is not life-threatening.

9) Is shingles contagious?

- No, shingles itself is not contagious but to a person who is not immune to chickenpox. Contact with the virus will give the person affected chickenpox.

10) Can shingles be contracted from someone with chickenpox?

- No, shingles cannot be contracted from someone with chickenpox.

11) What virus causes chickenpox?

- The varicella zoster virus causes chickenpox.

12) What are retroviruses?

- Retroviruses are viruses that are made of RNA.

13) Is Varicella a DNA virus or an RNA virus?

- Varicella is a DNA virus.

14) What is the abbreviation DNA?

- The abbreviation DNA is deoxyribonucleic acid.

15) What is the abbreviation RNA?

- The abbreviation RNA is ribonucleic acid.

16) Do all people who have had chicken pox also will have shingles?

- No, not all people who have had chicken pox will have shingles.

Section 3

1) What happens to the virus after a person recovers from chickenpox infection?

- After a person recovers from chickenpox infection, the virus stays in the body in a dormant phase.

2) Can the dormant virus in a person that recovers from chickenpox be reactivated?

- Yes, the dormant virus in a person that recovers from chickenpox can be reactivated.

3) What does the reactivated virus cause?

- The reactivated virus causes shingles.

4) Where does chickenpox stay in the body after treatment?

- Chickenpox stays dormant in the nerve tissue.

5) What is the function of a nerve?

- A nerve enables the transmission of electrical impulses.

6) Is chickenpox contagious?

-    Yes, chickenpox is contagious.

7) Can shingles affect internal organs?

-    Yes, shingles can affect internal organs.

8) The blisters in shingles are filled with?

-    The blisters in shingles are filled with pus.

9) How long does it take for shingles blisters to dry up?

-    Normally, it takes about one week to ten days for shingles blisters to dry up.

10) Does the pain usually go away when the blisters heal?

-    Yes, the pain usually goes away when the blisters heal.

11) Can blisters sometimes leave scars after they heal?

-    Yes, blisters can sometimes leave scars after they heal.

Section 4

1) Is chickenpox a classic disease for children?

- Yes, chickenpox is a classic disease for children.

2) Are the pustules contagious?

- Yes, the pustules are contagious.

3) What are the signs and symptoms of shingles?

- The signs and symptoms of shingles are pain, itching, red rash, burning, tingling, blisters, fatigue, light sensitivity, fever, etc.

4) What are the complications of shingles?

- The complications of shingles include infections, eye problems, vision loss, postherpetic neuralgia, neurological problems, facial paralysis, etc.

5) What is ophthalmic shingles?

- Ophthalmic shingles is shingles of the eye or around the eye.

6) Are eye problems caused by shingles an emergency?

- Yes, eye problems caused by shingles is an emergency.

7) Why are eye problems caused by shingles an emergency?

- Eye problems caused by shingles is an emergency because if not quickly treated, eye problems can lead to blindness.

8) What is the function of the optic nerve?

- The optic nerve transmits signals from the eye to the brain.

9) What is encephalitis?

- Encephalitis is the inflammation of the brain.

10) What is postherpetic neuralgia?

- Postherpetic neuralgia is prolonged shingles pain even after the blisters have healed.

11) What is the cause of postherpetic neuralgia?

- The cause of postherpetic neuralgia is due to damaged nerves.

Section 5

1) Can postherpetic neuralgia last for years?

-   Yes, postherpetic neuralgia can last for years.

2) Does post-herpetic neuralgia get worse with age?

-   Yes, post-herpetic neuralgia gets worse with age.

3) Could meningitis be a complication of shingles?

-   Yes, meningitis could be a complication of shingles.

4) What is meningitis?

-   Meningitis is the inflammation of the meninges.

5) What are meninges?

-   Meninges are membranes that protect the brain and spinal cord.

6) What is myalgia?

- Myalgia is muscle pain.

7) Could pneumonia be a complication of shingles?

- Yes, pneumonia could be a complication of shingles.

8) What is pneumonia?

- Pneumonia is the inflammation of alveoli.

9) What is the function of alveoli?

- Alveoli permit the exchange of gas during respiration.

Section 6

1) Could shingles lead to hepatitis?

- Yes, shingles could lead to hepatitis.

2) What is hepatitis?

- Hepatitis is the inflammation of the liver.

3) What are the risk factors for shingles?

- The risk factors for shingles include age, over 50 years, diseases that weaken the body's immune system, medications that weaken the immune system, stress, etc.

4) What are some diseases that weaken the immune system?

- Diseases like HIV and cancers can weaken the immune system.

5) Does the immune system function become less effective with age?

- Yes, the immune system function becomes less effective with age.

6) What are antigens?

- Antigens are substances that cause the body to activate the immune system.

7) What are examples of antigens?

- Examples of antigens include virus, bacteria, toxins, etc.

8) Antigens can also be called?

- Antigens can also be called immunogens.

9) Can physical exercise improve the immune system?

- Yes, physical exercise can improve the immune system.

10) Can psychological stress suppress the immune system?

- Yes, psychological stress can suppress the immune system.

Section 7

1) Can retinitis lead to blindness?

- Yes, retinitis can lead to blindness.

2) Can glaucoma lead to vision loss?

- Yes, glaucoma can lead to vision loss.

3) What is glaucoma?

- Glaucoma is the damage to the optic nerve.

4) What is retinitis?

- Retinitis is the inflammation of the retina.

5) What is the function of the retina?

- The retina is sensitive to light and sends this signal to the brain.

6) What is conjunctivitis?

- Conjunctivitis is the inflammation of the conjunctiva.

7) What is the conjunctiva?

- The conjunctiva is a transparent membrane that covers the sclera and inside the eyelids.

8) What is scleritis?

- Scleritis is the inflammation of the sclera.

9) What is the sclera?

- The sclera is the white part of the eye.

10) What is episcleritis?

- Episcleritis is the inflammation of the episclera.

11) What is the episclera?

- The episclera is the thin membrane that covers the sclera.

12) What is keratitis?

- Keratitis is the inflammation of the cornea.

Section 8

1) What is necrosis?

- Necrosis is the death of tissue in the body.

2) What causes necrosis?

- Necrosis is caused by an insufficient supply of oxygen and blood to a tissue or organ.

3) What is erythema?

- Erythema is redness of the skin due to inflammation.

4) What is prodrome?

- Prodrome is an early symptom or sign of a disease or illness.

5) Does shingles present the same symptoms in everybody?

- No, shingles does not always present the same symptoms in everybody.

6) What is vasculitis?

- Vasculitis is the inflammation of blood vessels.

7) Vasculitis is also called?

- Vasculitis is also called angiitis.

8) What are the kinds of blood vessels?

- The kinds of blood vessels are the arteries, the veins, and the capillaries.

9) What is the function of arteries?

- Arteries carry blood rich in oxygen from the heart.

10) What are arterioles?

- Arterioles are small arteries that lead to capillaries.

Section 9

1) What is the function of capillaries?

- Capillaries channel blood between the arterioles and venules.

2) What are the smallest blood vessels in the body?

- Capillaries are the smallest blood vessels in the body.

3) What are venules?

- Venules are small blood vessels that take blood from capillaries to veins.

4) What is the function of veins?

- Veins return blood to the heart.

5) What is a dermatome?

- A dermatome is an area of the skin connected to a single spinal nerve root.

6) What is an enzyme?

- An enzyme is a protein that speeds up
chemical reactions in the body.

Section 10

1) What is Ramsay Hunt syndrome?

- Ramsay Hunt syndrome is the paralysis of the facial nerve.

2) Ramsay Hunt syndrome is also known as?

- Ramsay Hunt syndrome is also known as herpes zoster oticus.

3) What is Herpes Zoster Oticus?

- Herpes Zoster Oticus is shingles infection of the ear.

4) Can Ramsay Hunt syndrome lead to hearing loss?

- Yes, Ramsay Hunt syndrome can lead to hearing loss.

5) Can shingles affect all parts of the ear?

- Yes, shingles can affect all parts of the ear.

6) What is tinnitus?

-    Tinnitus is the ringing in the ears.

Conclusion

Thank you again for purchasing this book. I hope it has helped you in your journey to understanding shingles and how it affects the body.

Please, if you enjoyed this book, I would like you to rate and comment. It'd be appreciated.

Thank you.